THE POWER OF GRATITUDE JORNAL

The 90-Day Gratitude Journal

A MINDFUL PRACTICE for Lifetime of HAPPINESS

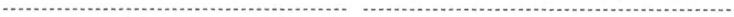

THE POWER OF GRATITUDE JORNAL

Creating an attitude of gratitude is probably the least demanding advance we can take to improve our lives· The joy that we make for ourselves by indicating our gratefulness has sweeping impacts, both for ourselves and for those we come into contact with· The potential for the appreciation to spread past those individuals likewise increments essentially – it tends to be profoundly infectious·

"At times, our own light goes out and is rekindled by a spark from another person. Each of us has cause to think with deep gratitude of those who have lighted the flame within us." – Albert Schweitzer

Well-Being: Appreciative individuals report more elevated levels of positive feelings, life fulfillment, essentialness, hopefulness and lower levels of sorrow and stress· The aura toward appreciation seems to improve charming inclination states more than it reduces undesirable feelings· Thankful individuals don't deny or overlook the negative parts of life·

DAY 1

DATE_____/_____/_____

> *When you are grateful, fear disappears and abundance appears.*
> — TONY ROBBINS

QUESTION #1: "I am grateful for_____, because _____."

_____

_____

_____

QUESTION #2: "What am I looking forward to today (or tomorrow)?"

_____

_____

_____

QUESTION #3: Describe your happiest childhood memory.

_____

_____

_____

_____

_____

_____

_____

_____

_____

DAY 2

DATE_____/_____/_____

Act with kindness, but do not expect gratitude.

— CONFUCIUS

QUESTION #1: "I am grateful for_____, because _____."

_____

_____

_____

QUESTION #2: "What am I looking forward to today (or tomorrow)?"

_____

_____

_____

QUESTION #3: What is a popular song that you enjoy (and why do you like it)?

_____

_____

_____

_____

_____

_____

_____

_____

DAY 3

DATE_____/_____/_____

> *Develop an attitude of gratitude. Say thank you to everyone you meet for everything they do for you.*
>
> — BRIAN TRACY

QUESTION #1: "I am grateful for_____, because _____."

_____

_____

_____

QUESTION #2: "What am I looking forward to today (or tomorrow)?"

_____

_____

_____

QUESTION #3: What is one of your favorite songs from your childhood?

_____

_____

_____

_____

_____

_____

_____

DAY 4

DATE_____/_____/_____

> ## An attitude of gratitude brings great things.
> — YOGI BHAJAN

QUESTION #1: "I am grateful for_____, because _____."

_____

_____

_____

QUESTION #2: "What am I looking forward to today (or tomorrow)?"

_____

_____

_____

QUESTION #3: Who is the one friend you can always rely on?

_____

_____

_____

_____

_____

_____

_____

_____

_____

DAY 5

DATE_____/_____/_____

Stop now. Enjoy the moment. It's now or never.

— MAXIME LAGACÉ

QUESTION #1: "I am grateful for_____, because _____."

_____

_____

_____

QUESTION #2: "What am I looking forward to today (or tomorrow)?"

_____

_____

_____

QUESTION #3: What is the biggest accomplishment in your personal life?

_____

_____

_____

_____

_____

_____

_____

_____

DAY 6

DATE____/____/____

> *When gratitude becomes an essential foundation in our lives,*
> *miracles start to appear everywhere.*
> — EMMANUEL DALGHER

QUESTION #1: "I am grateful for_____, because _____."

_____

_____

_____

QUESTION #2: "What am I looking forward to today (or tomorrow)?"

_____

_____

_____

QUESTION #3: What is the biggest accomplishment in your professional life?

_____

_____

_____

_____

_____

_____

_____

_____

DAY 7

DATE_____/_____/_____

> ## *The essence of all beautiful art is gratitude.*
> — FRIEDRICH NIETZCHE

QUESTION #1: "I am grateful for_____, because _____."

_____

_____

_____

QUESTION #2: "What am I looking forward to today (or tomorrow)?"

_____

_____

_____

QUESTION #3: What is your favorite memory of your father (or stepfather)?

_____

_____

_____

_____

_____

_____

_____

_____

DAY 8

DATE_____/_____/_____

> ## The smallest act of kindness is worth more than the grandest intention.
>
> — OSCAR WILDE

QUESTION #1: "I am grateful for_____, because _____."

_____

_____

_____

QUESTION #2: "What am I looking forward to today (or tomorrow)?"

_____

_____

_____

QUESTION #3: What is your favorite memory of your mother (or stepmother)?

_____

_____

_____

_____

_____

_____

_____

_____

DAY 9

No duty is more urgent than that of returning thanks.
— JAMES ALLEN

QUESTION #1: "I am grateful for_____, because _____."

_____

_____

_____

QUESTION #2: "What am I looking forward to today (or tomorrow)?"

_____

_____

_____

QUESTION #3: Describe your favorite pet (or former pet)?

_____

_____

_____

_____

_____

_____

_____

_____

_____

DAY 10

> *Gratitude changes everything.*
>
> — ANONYMOUS

QUESTION #1: "I am grateful for_____, because _____."

_____

_____

_____

QUESTION #2: "What am I looking forward to today (or tomorrow)?"

_____

_____

_____

QUESTION #3: List 10 hobbies and activities that bring you joy?

_____

_____

_____

_____

_____

_____

_____

_____

_____

DAY 11

DATE_____/_____/_____

> *Gratitude makes sense of your past, brings peace for today, and creates a vision for tomorrow.*
>
> — MELODY BEATTIE

QUESTION #1: "I am grateful for_____, because _____."

_____

_____

_____

QUESTION #2: "What am I looking forward to today (or tomorrow)?"

_____

_____

_____

QUESTION #3: What is a mistake that you've made and that ultimately led to a positive experience?

_____

_____

_____

_____

_____

_____

_____

_____

DAY 12

DATE_____/_____/_____

> *The highest tribute to the dead is not grief but gratitude.*
>
> — THORNTON WILDER

QUESTION #1: "I am grateful for_____, because _____."

_____

_____

_____

QUESTION #2: "What am I looking forward to today (or tomorrow)?"

_____

_____

_____

QUESTION #3: Describe a family tradition that you are most grateful for.

_____

_____

_____

_____

_____

_____

_____

_____

DAY 13

DATE_____/_____/_____

> *True forgiveness is when you can say, Thank you for that experience.*
> — OPRAH WINFREY

QUESTION #1: "I am grateful for_____, because _____."

_____

_____

_____

QUESTION #2: "What am I looking forward to today (or tomorrow)?"

_____

_____

_____

QUESTION #3: Who is a teacher or mentor that has made an impact on your life, and how did they help you?

_____

_____

_____

_____

_____

_____

_____

_____

DAY 14

DATE_____/_____/_____

> *Nothing new can come into your life unless you are grateful for what you already have.*
>
> — MICHAEL BERNHARD

QUESTION #1: "I am grateful for_____, because _____."

_____

_____

_____

QUESTION #2: "What am I looking forward to today (or tomorrow)?"

_____

_____

_____

QUESTION #3: What do you like the most about your town or city?

_____

_____

_____

_____

_____

_____

_____

_____

DAY 15

DATE_____/_____/_____

> *Appreciation is a wonderful thing: It makes what is excellent in others belong to us as well.*
>
> — VOLTAIRE

QUESTION #1: "I am grateful for_____, because _____."

_____

_____

_____

QUESTION #2: "What am I looking forward to today (or tomorrow)?"

_____

_____

_____

QUESTION #3: Describe your favorite location in your house and why you like it.

_____

_____

_____

_____

_____

_____

_____

_____

DAY 16

DATE_____/_____/_____

> ## There is always something to be grateful for.
> — ANONYMOUS

QUESTION #1: "I am grateful for_____, because _____."

_____

_____

_____

QUESTION #2: "What am I looking forward to today (or tomorrow)?"

_____

_____

_____

QUESTION #3: What is one thing you've learned this week that you're thankful for?

_____

_____

_____

_____

_____

_____

_____

_____

DAY 17

> *Nothing is more honorable than a grateful heart.*
> — LUCIUS ANNAEUS SENECA

QUESTION #1: "I am grateful for_____, because _____."

_____

_____

_____

QUESTION #2: "What am I looking forward to today (or tomorrow)?"

_____

_____

_____

QUESTION #3: Who made you smile in the past 24 hours and why?

_____

_____

_____

_____

_____

_____

_____

_____

DAY 18

DATE_____/_____/_____

> ## Gratitude; my cup over floweth.
>
> — OSCAR WILDE

QUESTION #1: "I am grateful for_____, because _____."

_____

_____

_____

QUESTION #2: "What am I looking forward to today (or tomorrow)?"

_____

_____

_____

QUESTION #3: What is a recent purchase that has added value to your life?

_____

_____

_____

_____

_____

_____

_____

_____

DAY 19

DATE_____/_____/_____

> ## *Hope has a good memory, gratitude a bad one.*
> — BALTASAR GRACIAN

QUESTION #1: "I am grateful for_____, because _____."

_____

_____

_____

QUESTION #2: "What am I looking forward to today (or tomorrow)?"

_____

_____

_____

QUESTION #3: What is biggest lesson you learned in child-hood?

_____

_____

_____

_____

_____

_____

_____

DAY 20

DATE____/____/____

> *There are always flowers for those who want to see them.*
>
> — HENRI MATISSE

QUESTION #1: "I am grateful for_____, because _____."

_____

_____

_____

QUESTION #2: "What am I looking forward to today (or tomorrow)?"

_____

_____

_____

QUESTION #3: List 10 ways you can share your gratitude with other people in the next 24 hours.

_____

_____

_____

_____

_____

_____

_____

_____

DAY 21

DATE_____/_____/_____

QUESTION #1: "I am grateful for_____, because _____."

_____

_____

_____

QUESTION #2: "What am I looking forward to today (or tomorrow)?"

_____

_____

_____

QUESTION #3: Describe your favorite smell.

_____

_____

_____

_____

_____

_____

_____

_____

DAY 22

DATE_____/_____/_____

> *Living in a state of gratitude is the gateway to grace.*
>
> — ARIANNA HUFFINGTON

QUESTION #1: "I am grateful for_____, because _____."

_____

_____

_____

QUESTION #2: "What am I looking forward to today (or tomorrow)?"

_____

_____

_____

QUESTION #3: Describe your favorite sound.

_____

_____

_____

_____

_____

_____

_____

_____

_____

DAY 23

My day begins and ends with gratitude.

— LOUISE HAY

QUESTION #1: "I am grateful for_____, because _____."

_____

_____

_____

QUESTION #2: "What am I looking forward to today (or tomorrow)?"

_____

_____

_____

QUESTION #3: Describe your favorite sight.

_____

_____

_____

_____

_____

_____

_____

_____

_____

DAY 24

> ## *Walk as if you are kissing the earth with your feet.*
> — THICH NHAT HANH

QUESTION #1: "I am grateful for_____, because _____."

_____

_____

_____

QUESTION #2: "What am I looking forward to today (or tomorrow)?"

_____

_____

_____

QUESTION #3: Describe your favorite taste.

_____

_____

_____

_____

_____

_____

_____

_____

_____

DAY 25

DATE_____/_____/_____

> *Things must be felt with the heart.*
>
> — HELEN KELLER

QUESTION #1: "I am grateful for_____, because _____."

_____

_____

_____

QUESTION #2: "What am I looking forward to today (or tomorrow)?"

_____

_____

_____

QUESTION #3: Describe your favorite sensation.

_____

_____

_____

_____

_____

_____

_____

_____

DAY 26

DATE_____/_____/_____

> *Forget injuries, never forget kindnesses.*
>
> — CONFUCIUS

QUESTION #1: "I am grateful for_____, because _____."

_____

_____

_____

QUESTION #2: "What am I looking forward to today (or tomorrow)?"

_____

_____

_____

QUESTION #3: How can you pamper yourself in the next 24 hours?

_____

_____

_____

_____

_____

_____

_____

DAY 27

DATE_____/_____/_____

> *Thank you is the best prayer that anyone could say. I say that one a lot. Thank you expresses extreme gratitude, humility, understanding.*
>
> — ALICE WALKER

QUESTION #1: "I am grateful for_____, because _____."

_____

_____

_____

QUESTION #2: "What am I looking forward to today (or tomorrow)?"

_____

_____

_____

QUESTION #3: Name and write about someone you've never met but who has helped your life in some way.

_____

_____

_____

_____

_____

_____

_____

_____

DAY 28

> *Gratitude is the fairest blossom that springs from the soul.*
>
> — HENRY WARD BEECHER

QUESTION #1: "I am grateful for_____, because _____."

_____

_____

_____

QUESTION #2: "What am I looking forward to today (or tomorrow)?"

_____

_____

_____

QUESTION #3: How is your life more positive today than it was a year ago?

_____

_____

_____

_____

_____

_____

_____

_____

DAY 29

DATE_____/_____/_____

> *Gratitude is riches. Complaint is poverty.*
>
> — DORIS DAY

QUESTION #1: "I am grateful for_____, because _____."

_____

_____

_____

QUESTION #2: "What am I looking forward to today (or tomorrow)?"

_____

_____

_____

QUESTION #3: What do other people like about you?

_____

_____

_____

_____

_____

_____

_____

_____

DAY 30

> So much has been given to me; I have no time to ponder over that which has been denied.
>
> — HELEN KELLER

QUESTION #1: "I am grateful for_____, because _____."

_____

_____

_____

QUESTION #2: "What am I looking forward to today (or tomorrow)?"

_____

_____

_____

QUESTION #3: List 10 skills you have that most people don't possess.

_____

_____

_____

_____

_____

_____

_____

_____

_____

DAY 31

DATE_____/_____/_____

> *There is so much to be grateful for, just open your eyes.*
>
> — ANONYMOUS

QUESTION #1: "I am grateful for_____, because _____."

_____

_____

_____

QUESTION #2: "What am I looking forward to today (or tomorrow)?"

_____

_____

_____

QUESTION #3: Describe the last time someone helped you solve a problem at work.

_____

_____

_____

_____

_____

_____

_____

_____

DAY 32

> ## *If you want to find happiness, find gratitude.*
> — STEVE MARABOLI

QUESTION #1: "I am grateful for_____, because _____."

_____

_____

_____

QUESTION #2: "What am I looking forward to today (or tomorrow)?"

_____

_____

_____

QUESTION #3: What is your favorite part of your daily routine?

_____

_____

_____

_____

_____

_____

_____

_____

DAY 33

DATE_____/_____/_____

QUESTION #1: "I am grateful for_____, because _____."

_____

_____

_____

QUESTION #2: "What am I looking forward to today (or tomorrow)?"

_____

_____

_____

QUESTION #3: What is a great book you've recently read?

_____

_____

_____

_____

_____

_____

_____

_____

_____

DAY 34

> *The roots of all goodness lie in the soil of appreciation for goodness.*
>
> — DALAI LAMA

QUESTION #1: "I am grateful for_____, because _____."

_____

_____

_____

QUESTION #2: "What am I looking forward to today (or tomorrow)?"

_____

_____

_____

QUESTION #3: What is your favorite holiday, and why do you love it?

_____

_____

_____

_____

_____

_____

_____

_____

DAY 35

> *Gratitude is the sign of noble souls.*
>
> — AESOP

QUESTION #1: "I am grateful for_____, because _____."

_____

_____

_____

QUESTION #2: "What am I looking forward to today (or tomorrow)?"

_____

_____

_____

QUESTION #3: What is your favorite TV show, and why do you love it?

_____

_____

_____

_____

_____

_____

_____

_____

DAY 36

> *Every blessing ignored becomes a curse.*
>
> — PAULO COELHO

QUESTION #1: "I am grateful for_____, because _____."

_____

_____

_____

QUESTION #2: "What am I looking forward to today (or tomorrow)?"

_____

_____

_____

QUESTION #3: What is your favorite movie, and why do you love it?

_____

_____

_____

_____

_____

_____

_____

_____

DAY 37

DATE_____/_____/_____

> *Through the eyes of gratitude, everything is a miracle.*
> — MARY DAVIS

QUESTION #1: "I am grateful for_____, because _____."

_____

_____

_____

QUESTION #2: "What am I looking forward to today (or tomorrow)?"

_____

_____

_____

QUESTION #3: What is your favorite way to enjoy nature (e.g., walking in the woods, sitting on the beach, hiking in the mountains, etc.)?

_____

_____

_____

_____

_____

_____

_____

DAY 38

DATE_____/_____/_____

> *This a wonderful day. I've never seen this one before.*
>
> — MAYA ANGELOU

QUESTION #1: "I am grateful for_____, because _____."

_____

_____

_____

QUESTION #2: "What am I looking forward to today (or tomorrow)?"

_____

_____

_____

QUESTION #3: Write about a recent obstacle you faced and how you overcame it.

_____

_____

_____

_____

_____

_____

_____

_____

DAY 39

> *The real gift of gratitude is that the more grateful you are,*
> *the more present you become.*
>
> — ROBERT HOLDEN

QUESTION #1: "I am grateful for_____, because _____."

_____

_____

_____

QUESTION #2: "What am I looking forward to today (or tomorrow)?"

_____

_____

_____

QUESTION #3: Describe a favorite pet and what you love(d)
about it.

_____

_____

_____

_____

_____

_____

_____

_____

DAY 40

DATE____/____/____

> *If you are really thankful, what do you do? You share.*
>
> — W. CLEMENT STONE

QUESTION #1: "I am grateful for_____, because _____."

_____

_____

_____

QUESTION #2: "What am I looking forward to today (or tomorrow)?"

_____

_____

_____

QUESTION #3: List 10 things you are looking forward to in the next year.

_____

_____

_____

_____

_____

_____

_____

_____

_____

DAY 41

DATE_____/_____/_____

> *Three meals plus bedtime make four sure blessings a day.*
> — MASON COOLEY

QUESTION #1: "I am grateful for_____, because _____."

_____

_____

_____

QUESTION #2: "What am I looking forward to today (or tomorrow)?"

_____

_____

_____

QUESTION #3: What do you love most about your country?

_____

_____

_____

_____

_____

_____

_____

_____

_____

DAY 42

> *Gratitude is the most exquisite form of courtesy.*
>
> — JACQUES MARITAIN

QUESTION #1: "I am grateful for_____, because _____."

_____

_____

_____

QUESTION #2: "What am I looking forward to today (or tomorrow)?"

_____

_____

_____

QUESTION #3: What is your favorite food you love to indulge in?

_____

_____

_____

_____

_____

_____

_____

_____

DAY 43

The struggle ends when gratitude begins.

— NEALE DONALD WALSCH

QUESTION #1: "I am grateful for_____, because _____."

_____

_____

_____

QUESTION #2: "What am I looking forward to today (or tomorrow)?"

_____

_____

_____

QUESTION #3: Write about someone who makes your life better.

_____

_____

_____

_____

_____

_____

_____

_____

_____

DAY 44

> *When we give cheerfully and accept gratefully, everyone is blessed.*
>
> — MAYA ANGELOU

QUESTION #1: "I am grateful for_____, because _____."

_____

_____

_____

QUESTION #2: "What am I looking forward to today (or tomorrow)?"

_____

_____

_____

QUESTION #3: If you're single, what is your favorite part about being single? Or if you're married, what is your favorite part about being married?

_____

_____

_____

_____

_____

_____

_____

DAY 45

> ## Don't pray when it rains if you don't pray when the sun shines.
> — LEROY SATCHEL PAIGE

QUESTION #1: "I am grateful for_____, because _____."

_____

_____

_____

QUESTION #2: "What am I looking forward to today (or tomorrow)?"

_____

_____

_____

QUESTION #3: What is today's weather, and what is one positive thing you can say about it?

_____

_____

_____

_____

_____

_____

_____

_____

DAY 46

DATE_____/_____/_____

> *Gratitude opens the door to the power, the wisdom, the creativity of the universe. You open the door through gratitude.*
>
> — DEEPAK CHOPRA

QUESTION #1: "I am grateful for_____, because _____."

_____

_____

_____

QUESTION #2: "What am I looking forward to today (or tomorrow)?"

_____

_____

_____

QUESTION #3: Describe a weird family tradition that you love.

_____

_____

_____

_____

_____

_____

_____

_____

DAY 47

DATE_____ / _____ / _____

> ## May you wake with gratitude.
> — ANONYMOUS

QUESTION #1: "I am grateful for_____, because _____."

_____

_____

_____

QUESTION #2: "What am I looking forward to today (or tomorrow)?"

_____

_____

_____

QUESTION #3: When was the last time you had a genuine belly laugh, and why was it so funny?

_____

_____

_____

_____

_____

_____

_____

_____

DAY 48

DATE_____/_____/_____

> *Our favorite attitude should be gratitude.*
>
> — ZIG ZIGLAR

QUESTION #1: "I am grateful for_____, because _____."

_____

_____

_____

QUESTION #2: "What am I looking forward to today (or tomorrow)?"

_____

_____

_____

QUESTION #3: What body part or organ are you most grateful for today (e.g., your eyes because you got to see a new movie)?

_____

_____

_____

_____

_____

_____

_____

DAY 49

Gratitude turns what we have into enough.

— AESOP

QUESTION #1: "I am grateful for_____, because _____."

_____

_____

_____

QUESTION #2: "What am I looking forward to today (or tomorrow)?"

_____

_____

_____

QUESTION #3: What is a major lesson that you learned from your job?

_____

_____

_____

_____

_____

_____

_____

_____

DAY 50

> *Reflect upon your present blessings, of which every man has plenty; not on your past misfortunes, of which all men have some.*
>
> — CHARLES DICKENS

QUESTION #1: "I am grateful for_____, because _____."

_____

_____

_____

QUESTION #2: "What am I looking forward to today (or tomorrow)?"

_____

_____

_____

QUESTION #3: List 10 items that you take for granted and that might not be available to people in other parts of the world (e.g., clean water, electricity, etc.).

_____

_____

_____

_____

_____

_____

_____

DAY 51

DATE_____/_____/_____

> *He is a wise man who does not grieve for the things which he has not, but rejoices for those which he has.*
>
> — EPICTETUS

QUESTION #1: "I am grateful for_____, because _____."

_____

_____

_____

QUESTION #2: "What am I looking forward to today (or tomorrow)?"

_____

_____

_____

QUESTION #3: Write about a recent time when a stranger did something nice for you.

_____

_____

_____

_____

_____

_____

_____

_____

DAY 52

DATE_____/_____/_____

> *Find the good and praise it.*
>
> — ALEX HALEY

QUESTION #1: "I am grateful for_____, because _____."

_____

_____

_____

QUESTION #2: "What am I looking forward to today (or tomorrow)?"

_____

_____

_____

QUESTION #3: What is the hardest thing you've had to do which led to a major personal accomplishment?

_____

_____

_____

_____

_____

_____

_____

_____

DAY 53

DATE_____ / _____ / _____

> *A moment of gratitude makes a difference in your attitude.*
>
> — BRUCE WILKINSON

QUESTION #1: "I am grateful for_____, because _____."

_____

_____

_____

QUESTION #2: "What am I looking forward to today (or tomorrow)?"

_____

_____

_____

QUESTION #3: What is one aspect about your health that you're grateful for?

_____

_____

_____

_____

_____

_____

_____

DAY 54

> *What separates privilege from entitlement is gratitude.*
>
> — BRENÉ BROWN

QUESTION #1: "I am grateful for_____, because _____."

_____

_____

_____

QUESTION #2: "What am I looking forward to today (or tomorrow)?"

_____

_____

_____

QUESTION #3: Who can you count on whenever you need someone to talk to and why?

_____

_____

_____

_____

_____

_____

_____

_____

DAY 55

DATE____/____/____

The more grateful I am, the more beauty I see.

—MARY DAVIS

QUESTION #1: "I am grateful for_____, because _____."

_____

_____

_____

QUESTION #2: "What am I looking forward to today (or tomorrow)?"

_____

_____

_____

QUESTION #3: Describe the last time you procrastinated on a task that wasn't as difficult as you thought it would be.

_____

_____

_____

_____

_____

_____

_____

_____

DAY 56

DATE_____/_____/_____

> *When it comes to life the critical thing is whether you take things for granted or take them with gratitude.*
>
> — G.K. CHESTERTON

QUESTION #1: "I am grateful for_____, because _____."

_____

_____

_____

QUESTION #2: "What am I looking forward to today (or tomorrow)?"

_____

_____

_____

QUESTION #3: What is your favorite habit, and why it is an important part of your daily routine?

_____

_____

_____

_____

_____

_____

_____

DAY 57

DATE_____/_____/_____

> *It is not joy that makes us grateful,
> it is gratitude that makes us joyful.*
>
> — DAVID STEINDL-RAST

QUESTION #1: "I am grateful for_____, because _____."

_____

_____

_____

QUESTION #2: "What am I looking forward to today (or tomorrow)?"

_____

_____

_____

QUESTION #3: Describe a "perfect day" that you recently had.

_____

_____

_____

_____

_____

_____

_____

_____

DAY 58

> *Gratitude and attitude are not challenges; they are choices.*
> — ROBERT BRAATHE

QUESTION #1: "I am grateful for_____, because _____."

_____

_____

_____

QUESTION #2: "What am I looking forward to today (or tomorrow)?"

_____

_____

_____

QUESTION #3: What is a favorite country that you've visited?

_____

_____

_____

_____

_____

_____

_____

_____

_____

DAY 59

DATE_____/_____/_____

> *We must never forget the importance of gratitude.*
>
> — ANONYMOUS

QUESTION #1: "I am grateful for_____, because _____."

_____

_____

_____

QUESTION #2: "What am I looking forward to today (or tomorrow)?"

_____

_____

_____

QUESTION #3: Describe a funny YouTube video that you recently watched.

_____

_____

_____

_____

_____

_____

_____

_____

DAY 60

> *Gratitude is not only the greatest of virtues but the parent of all others.*
>
> — CICERO

QUESTION #1: "I am grateful for_____, because _____."

_____

_____

_____

QUESTION #2: "What am I looking forward to today (or tomorrow)?"

_____

_____

_____

QUESTION #3: List 10 qualities you like about yourself.

_____

_____

_____

_____

_____

_____

_____

_____

_____

_____

DAY 61

DATE____/____/____

> *Feeling gratitude and not expressing it is like wrapping a present and not giving it.*
>
> — WILLIAM ARTHUR WARD

QUESTION #1: "I am grateful for_____, because _____."

_____

_____

_____

QUESTION #2: "What am I looking forward to today (or tomorrow)?"

_____

_____

_____

QUESTION #3: What is one thing you look forward to enjoying each day after work?

_____

_____

_____

_____

_____

_____

_____

_____

DAY 62

DATE_____/_____/_____

What are you grateful for today?

QUESTION #1: "I am grateful for_____, because _____."

_____

_____

_____

QUESTION #2: "What am I looking forward to today (or tomorrow)?"

_____

_____

_____

QUESTION #3: What was something you did for the first time recently?

_____

_____

_____

_____

_____

_____

_____

_____

DAY 63

DATE_____/_____/_____

> *We must find time to stop and thank the people*
> *who make a difference in our lives.*
>
> — JOHN F. KENNEDY

QUESTION #1: "I am grateful for_____, because _____."

_____

_____

_____

QUESTION #2: "What am I looking forward to today (or tomorrow)?"

_____

_____

_____

QUESTION #3: What is what one lesson you have learned from rude people?

_____

_____

_____

_____

_____

_____

_____

_____

DAY 64

DATE_____/_____/_____

> *Wear gratitude like a cloak and it will feed every corner of your life.*
>
> — RUMI

QUESTION #1: "I am grateful for_____, because _____."

_____

_____

_____

QUESTION #2: "What am I looking forward to today (or tomorrow)?"

_____

_____

_____

QUESTION #3: When was the last time you had a great nap where you awoke feeling fully refreshed?

_____

_____

_____

_____

_____

_____

_____

_____

DAY 65

DATE_____/_____/_____

> *May the work of your hands be a sign of gratitude and reverence to the human condition.*
>
> — MAHATMA GANDHI

QUESTION #1: "I am grateful for_____, because _____."

_____

_____

_____

QUESTION #2: "What am I looking forward to today (or tomorrow)?"

_____

_____

_____

QUESTION #3: Shower or bath? Which do you prefer and why?

_____

_____

_____

_____

_____

_____

_____

_____

DAY 66

DATE_____/_____/_____

> *The deepest craving of human nature is the need to be appreciated.*
> — WILLIAM JAMES

QUESTION #1: "I am grateful for_____, because _____."

_____

_____

_____

QUESTION #2: "What am I looking forward to today (or tomorrow)?"

_____

_____

_____

QUESTION #3: Write about a time where you felt courageous.

_____

_____

_____

_____

_____

_____

_____

_____

DAY 67

DATE____/____/____

> ## *If you have lived, take thankfully the past.*
> — JOHN DRYDEN

QUESTION #1: "I am grateful for_____, because _____."

_____

_____

_____

QUESTION #2: "What am I looking forward to today (or tomorrow)?"

_____

_____

_____

QUESTION #3: What are a few ways you can appreciate your health whenever you're sick?

_____

_____

_____

_____

_____

_____

_____

_____

DAY 68

> *It's a sign of mediocrity when you demonstrate gratitude with moderation.*
>
> — ROBERTO BENIGNI

QUESTION #1: "I am grateful for_____, because _____."

_____

_____

_____

QUESTION #2: "What am I looking forward to today (or tomorrow)?"

_____

_____

_____

QUESTION #3: What is a favorite drink that you like to enjoy each day?

_____

_____

_____

_____

_____

_____

_____

_____

DAY 69

DATE_____/_____/_____

QUESTION #1: "I am grateful for_____, because _____"

_____

_____

_____

QUESTION #2: "What am I looking forward to today (or tomorrow)?"

_____

_____

_____

QUESTION #3: Who has forgiven you for a mistake you've made in the past?

_____

_____

_____

_____

_____

_____

_____

DAY 70

> ## *Have an attitude of gratitude.*
> — THOMAS S. MONSON

QUESTION #1: "I am grateful for_____, because _____."

_____

_____

_____

QUESTION #2: "What am I looking forward to today (or tomorrow)?"

_____

_____

_____

QUESTION #3: List 10 things you have now that you didn't have five years ago.

_____

_____

_____

_____

_____

_____

_____

_____

DAY 71

DATE_____/_____/_____

> *When I started counting my blessings, my whole life turned around.*
> — WILLIE NELSON

QUESTION #1: "I am grateful for_____, because _____."

_____

_____

_____

QUESTION #2: "What am I looking forward to today (or tomorrow)?"

_____

_____

_____

QUESTION #3: What aspects of your job do you enjoy the most?

_____

_____

_____

_____

_____

_____

_____

_____

DAY 72

DATE_____/_____/_____

> *We often take for granted the very things that most deserve our gratitude.*
> — CYNTHIA OZICK

QUESTION #1: "I am grateful for_____, because _____."

_____

_____

_____

QUESTION #2: "What am I looking forward to today (or tomorrow)?"

_____

_____

_____

QUESTION #3: What is a positive aspect that you can learn from one of your negative qualities (e.g., being anxious means you're really good at planning things out)?

_____

_____

_____

_____

_____

_____

_____

DAY 73

> ## *Enough is a feast.*
> — BUDDHIST PROVERB

QUESTION #1: "I am grateful for_____, because _____."

_____

_____

_____

QUESTION #2: "What am I looking forward to today (or tomorrow)?"

_____

_____

_____

QUESTION #3: What are a few aspects of modern technology that you love?

_____

_____

_____

_____

_____

_____

_____

_____

DAY 74

> *The way to develop the best that is in a person is by appreciation and encouragement.*
>
> — CHARLES SCHWAB

QUESTION #1: "I am grateful for_____, because _____."

_____

_____

_____

QUESTION #2: "What am I looking forward to today (or tomorrow)?"

_____

_____

_____

QUESTION #3: What is a great recipe you've prepared that others rave about?

_____

_____

_____

_____

_____

_____

_____

_____

DAY 75

DATE____/____/____

> ## We can choose to be grateful no matter what.
> — DIETER F. UCHTDORF

QUESTION #1: "I am grateful for_____, because _____."

_____

_____

_____

QUESTION #2: "What am I looking forward to today (or tomorrow)?"

_____

_____

_____

QUESTION #3: Describe a recent time when you truly felt at peace.

_____

_____

_____

_____

_____

_____

_____

DAY 76

DATE_____/_____/_____

> *Let us be grateful to the people who make us happy; they are the charming gardeners who make our souls blossom.*
>
> — MARCEL PROUST

QUESTION #1: "I am grateful for_____, because _____."

_____

_____

_____

QUESTION #2: "What am I looking forward to today (or tomorrow)?"

_____

_____

_____

QUESTION #3: What is your favorite quote or bit of wisdom that you like to frequently share with others?

_____

_____

_____

_____

_____

_____

_____

_____

DAY 77

DATE_____/_____/_____

> *A sense of blessedness comes from a change of heart,*
> *not from more blessings.*
>
> — MASON COOLEY

QUESTION #1: "I am grateful for_____, because _____."

_____

_____

_____

QUESTION #2: "What am I looking forward to today (or tomorrow)?"

_____

_____

_____

QUESTION #3: What is your favorite sports team? Describe a
cherished memory you have when cheering for this team.

_____

_____

_____

_____

_____

_____

_____

_____

DAY 78

> ## The best way to pay for a lovely moment is to enjoy it.
> — RICHARD BACH

QUESTION #1: "I am grateful for_____, because _____."

_____

_____

_____

QUESTION #2: "What am I looking forward to today (or tomorrow)?"

_____

_____

_____

QUESTION #3: Are you a morning person or a night owl? What do you love most about this part of the day?

_____

_____

_____

_____

_____

_____

_____

_____

DAY 79

DATE____/____/____

> *Thankfulness may consist merely of words. Gratitude is shown in acts.*
>
> — HENRI FREDERIC AMIEL

QUESTION #1: "I am grateful for_____, because _____."

_____

_____

_____

QUESTION #2: "What am I looking forward to today (or tomorrow)?"

_____

_____

_____

QUESTION #3: What is the last thank you note you've re-
ceived, and why?

_____

_____

_____

_____

_____

_____

_____

_____

DAY 80

DATE_____/_____/_____

> *I was complaining that I had no shoes till I met a man who had no feet.*
>
> — CONFUCIUS

QUESTION #1: "I am grateful for_____, because _____."

_____

_____

_____

QUESTION #2: "What am I looking forward to today (or tomorrow)?"

_____

_____

_____

QUESTION #3: List 10 of your favorite possessions.

_____

_____

_____

_____

_____

_____

_____

_____

_____

_____

DAY 81

DATE_____/_____/_____

> *Giving is an expression of gratitude for our blessings.*
> — LAURA ARRILLAGA-ANDREESSEN

QUESTION #1: "I am grateful for_____, because _____."

_____

_____

_____

QUESTION #2: "What am I looking forward to today (or tomorrow)?"

_____

_____

_____

QUESTION #3: What is a small win that you accomplished in the past 24 hours?

_____

_____

_____

_____

_____

_____

_____

_____

DAY 82

> *Be grateful for what you have, and work hard for what you don't have.*
>
> — ANONYMOUS

QUESTION #1: "I am grateful for_____, because _____."

_____

_____

_____

QUESTION #2: "What am I looking forward to today (or tomorrow)?"

_____

_____

_____

QUESTION #3: Describe one thing that you like about your daily commute to work.

_____

_____

_____

_____

_____

_____

_____

_____

DAY 83

> ## *It is only with gratitude that life becomes rich.*
> — DEITRICH BONHEIFFER

QUESTION #1: "I am grateful for_____, because _____."

_____

_____

_____

QUESTION #2: "What am I looking forward to today (or tomorrow)?"

_____

_____

_____

QUESTION #3: What is a personal viewpoint that positively defines you as a person?

_____

_____

_____

_____

_____

_____

_____

_____

DAY 84

DATE_____/_____/_____

> ## We can complain because rose bushes have thorns, or rejoice because thorns have roses.
>
> — ALPHONSE KARR

QUESTION #1: "I am grateful for_____, because _____."

_____

_____

_____

QUESTION #2: "What am I looking forward to today (or tomorrow)?"

_____

_____

_____

QUESTION #3: Describe an experience that was painful but made you a stronger person.

_____

_____

_____

_____

_____

_____

_____

_____

DAY 85

DATE_____/_____/_____

QUESTION #1: "I am grateful for_____, because _____."

_____

_____

_____

QUESTION #2: "What am I looking forward to today (or tomorrow)?"

_____

_____

_____

QUESTION #3: What is your favorite season, and what do you like about it?

_____

_____

_____

_____

_____

_____

_____

_____

DAY 86

DATE_____/_____/_____

> *May the gratitude in my heart kiss all the universe.*
>
> — HAFIZ

QUESTION #1: "I am grateful for_____, because _____."

_____

_____

_____

QUESTION #2: "What am I looking forward to today (or tomorrow)?"

_____

_____

_____

QUESTION #3: What makes you beautiful?

_____

_____

_____

_____

_____

_____

_____

_____

_____

DAY 87

DATE_____/_____/_____

Humor is mankind's greatest blessing.

— MARK TWAIN

QUESTION #1: "I am grateful for_____, because _____."

_____

_____

_____

QUESTION #2: "What am I looking forward to today (or tomorrow)?"

_____

_____

_____

QUESTION #3: What are you most looking forward to this week?

_____

_____

_____

_____

_____

_____

_____

_____

DAY 88

DATE_____/_____/_____

> *Showing gratitude is one of the simplest yet most powerful things humans can do for each other.*
>
> — RANDY RAUSCH

QUESTION #1: "I am grateful for_____, because _____."

_____

_____

_____

QUESTION #2: "What am I looking forward to today (or tomorrow)?"

_____

_____

_____

QUESTION #3: What is an app or piece of technology that you use every day that adds value to your life?

_____

_____

_____

_____

_____

_____

_____

_____

DAY 89

DATE_____ / _____ / _____

> *If the only prayer you said in your whole life was "thank you" that would suffice.*
>
> — MEISTER ECKHART

QUESTION #1: "I am grateful for_____, because _____."

_____

_____

_____

QUESTION #2: "What am I looking forward to today (or tomorrow)?"

_____

_____

_____

QUESTION #3: What makes you happy to be alive?

_____

_____

_____

_____

_____

_____

_____

_____

_____

DAY 90

It's not happiness that brings us gratitude.
It's gratitude that brings us happiness.

— ANONYMOUS

QUESTION #1: "I am grateful for_____, because _____."

_____

_____

_____

QUESTION #2: "What am I looking forward to today (or tomorrow)?"

_____

_____

_____

QUESTION #3: List 10 things you like about your job or work-place.

_____

_____

_____

_____

_____

_____

_____

_____

_____

DATE_____/_____/_____

It's not happiness that brings us gratitude.
It's gratitude that brings us happiness.

— ANONYMOUS

QUESTION #1: "I am grateful for_____, because _____."

_____

_____

_____

QUESTION #2: "What am I looking forward to today (or tomorrow)?"

_____

_____

_____

QUESTION #3: List 10 things you like about your job or work-place.

_____

_____

_____

_____

_____

_____

_____

DATE_____/_____/_____

> ### *It's not happiness that brings us gratitude.*
> ### *It's gratitude that brings us happiness.*
> — ANONYMOUS

QUESTION #1: "I am grateful for_____, because _____."

_____

_____

_____

QUESTION #2: "What am I looking forward to today (or tomorrow)?"

_____

_____

_____

QUESTION #3: List 10 things you like about your job or work-place.

_____

_____

_____

_____

_____

_____

_____

DATE_____/_____/_____

It's not happiness that brings us gratitude.
It's gratitude that brings us happiness.

— ANONYMOUS

QUESTION #1: "I am grateful for_____, because _____."

_____

_____

_____

QUESTION #2: "What am I looking forward to today (or tomorrow)?"

_____

_____

_____

QUESTION #3: List 10 things you like about your job or work-place.

_____

_____

_____

_____

_____

_____

_____

DATE_____/_____/_____

> ### *It's not happiness that brings us gratitude.*
> ### *It's gratitude that brings us happiness.*
>
> — ANONYMOUS

QUESTION #1: "I am grateful for_____, because _____."

_____

_____

_____

QUESTION #2: "What am I looking forward to today (or tomorrow)?"

_____

_____

_____

QUESTION #3: List 10 things you like about your job or work-place.

_____

_____

_____

_____

_____

_____

_____

DATE_____/_____/_____

QUESTION #1: "I am grateful for_____, because _____."

_____

_____

_____

QUESTION #2: "What am I looking forward to today (or tomorrow)?"

_____

_____

_____

QUESTION #3: List 10 things you like about your job or work-place.

_____

_____

_____

_____

_____

_____

_____

_____

DATE____/____/____

> *It's not happiness that brings us gratitude.*
> *It's gratitude that brings us happiness.*
>
> — ANONYMOUS

QUESTION #1: "I am grateful for_____, because _____."

_____

_____

_____

QUESTION #2: "What am I looking forward to today (or tomorrow)?"

_____

_____

_____

QUESTION #3: List 10 things you like about your job or work-place.

_____

_____

_____

_____

_____

_____

_____

_____

DATE_____/_____/_____

> *It's not happiness that brings us gratitude.*
> *It's gratitude that brings us happiness.*
>
> — ANONYMOUS

QUESTION #1: "I am grateful for_____, because _____."

_____

_____

_____

QUESTION #2: "What am I looking forward to today (or tomorrow)?"

_____

_____

_____

QUESTION #3: List 10 things you like about your job or work-place.

_____

_____

_____

_____

_____

_____

_____

DATE_____/_____/_____

> *It's not happiness that brings us gratitude.*
> *It's gratitude that brings us happiness.*
>
> — ANONYMOUS

QUESTION #1: "I am grateful for_____, because _____."

_____

_____

_____

QUESTION #2: "What am I looking forward to today (or tomorrow)?"

_____

_____

_____

QUESTION #3: List 10 things you like about your job or work-place.

_____

_____

_____

_____

_____

_____

_____

_____

DATE_____/_____/_____

> ## *It's not happiness that brings us gratitude.*
> ## *It's gratitude that brings us happiness.*
>
> — ANONYMOUS

QUESTION #1: "I am grateful for_____, because _____."

_____

_____

_____

QUESTION #2: "What am I looking forward to today (or tomorrow)?"

_____

_____

_____

QUESTION #3: List 10 things you like about your job or work-place.

_____

_____

_____

_____

_____

_____

_____

DATE____/____/____

QUESTION #1: "I am grateful for_____, because _____."

_____

_____

_____

QUESTION #2: "What am I looking forward to today (or tomorrow)?"

_____

_____

_____

QUESTION #3: List 10 things you like about your job or work-place.

_____

_____

_____

_____

_____

_____

_____

_____

DATE_____/_____/_____

> ### *It's not happiness that brings us gratitude.*
> ### *It's gratitude that brings us happiness.*
>
> — ANONYMOUS

QUESTION #1: "I am grateful for_____, because _____."

_____

_____

_____

QUESTION #2: "What am I looking forward to today (or tomorrow)?"

_____

_____

_____

QUESTION #3: List 10 things you like about your job or work-place.

_____

_____

_____

_____

_____

_____

_____

_____

DATE_____/_____/_____

> ## *It's not happiness that brings us gratitude.*
> ## *It's gratitude that brings us happiness.*
> — ANONYMOUS

QUESTION #1: "I am grateful for_____, because _____."

_____

_____

_____

QUESTION #2: "What am I looking forward to today (or tomorrow)?"

_____

_____

_____

QUESTION #3: List 10 things you like about your job or work-place.

_____

_____

_____

_____

_____

_____

_____

_____

DATE_____/_____/_____

> ## *It's not happiness that brings us gratitude.*
> ## *It's gratitude that brings us happiness.*
>
> — ANONYMOUS

QUESTION #1: "I am grateful for_____, because _____."

_____

_____

_____

QUESTION #2: "What am I looking forward to today (or tomorrow)?"

_____

_____

_____

QUESTION #3: List 10 things you like about your job or work-place.

_____

_____

_____

_____

_____

_____

_____

DATE_____/_____/_____

> *It's not happiness that brings us gratitude.*
> *It's gratitude that brings us happiness.*
>
> — ANONYMOUS

QUESTION #1: "I am grateful for_____, because _____."

_____

_____

_____

QUESTION #2: "What am I looking forward to today (or tomorrow)?"

_____

_____

_____

QUESTION #3: List 10 things you like about your job or work-place.

_____

_____

_____

_____

_____

_____

_____

_____

DATE_____/_____/_____

> *It's not happiness that brings us gratitude.*
> *It's gratitude that brings us happiness.*
>
> — ANONYMOUS

QUESTION #1: "I am grateful for_____, because _____."

_____

_____

_____

QUESTION #2: "What am I looking forward to today (or tomorrow)?"

_____

_____

_____

QUESTION #3: List 10 things you like about your job or work-place.

_____

_____

_____

_____

_____

_____

_____

_____

DATE_____/_____/_____

> *It's not happiness that brings us gratitude.*
> *It's gratitude that brings us happiness.*
>
> — ANONYMOUS

QUESTION #1: "I am grateful for_____, because _____."

_____

_____

_____

QUESTION #2: "What am I looking forward to today (or tomorrow)?"

_____

_____

_____

QUESTION #3: List 10 things you like about your job or work-place.

_____

_____

_____

_____

_____

_____

_____

_____

DATE_____/_____/_____

> ## It's not happiness that brings us gratitude.
> ## It's gratitude that brings us happiness.
>
> — ANONYMOUS

QUESTION #1: "I am grateful for_____, because _____."

_____

_____

_____

QUESTION #2: "What am I looking forward to today (or tomorrow)?"

_____

_____

_____

QUESTION #3: List 10 things you like about your job or work-place.

_____

_____

_____

_____

_____

_____

_____

DATE_____/_____/_____

QUESTION #1: "I am grateful for_____, because _____."

_____

_____

_____

QUESTION #2: "What am I looking forward to today (or tomorrow)?"

_____

_____

_____

QUESTION #3: List 10 things you like about your job or work-place.

_____

_____

_____

_____

_____

_____

_____

_____

DATE_____/_____/_____

> ### *It's not happiness that brings us gratitude.*
> ### *It's gratitude that brings us happiness.*
>
> — ANONYMOUS

QUESTION #1: "I am grateful for_____, because _____."

_____

_____

_____

QUESTION #2: "What am I looking forward to today (or tomorrow)?"

_____

_____

_____

QUESTION #3: List 10 things you like about your job or work-place.

_____

_____

_____

_____

_____

_____

_____

_____

DATE_____/_____/_____

> *It's not happiness that brings us gratitude.*
> *It's gratitude that brings us happiness.*
>
> — ANONYMOUS

QUESTION #1: "I am grateful for_____, because _____."

_____

_____

_____

QUESTION #2: "What am I looking forward to today (or tomorrow)?"

_____

_____

_____

QUESTION #3: List 10 things you like about your job or work-place.

_____

_____

_____

_____

_____

_____

_____

DATE_____/_____/_____

QUESTION #1: "I am grateful for_____, because _____."

_____

_____

_____

QUESTION #2: "What am I looking forward to today (or tomorrow)?"

_____

_____

_____

QUESTION #3: List 10 things you like about your job or work-place.

_____

_____

_____

_____

_____

_____

_____

_____

DATE_____/_____/_____

> ## It's not happiness that brings us gratitude.
> ## It's gratitude that brings us happiness.
>
> — ANONYMOUS

QUESTION #1: "I am grateful for_____, because _____."

_____

_____

_____

QUESTION #2: "What am I looking forward to today (or tomorrow)?"

_____

_____

_____

QUESTION #3: List 10 things you like about your job or work-place.

_____

_____

_____

_____

_____

_____

_____

_____

DATE_____/_____/_____

> *It's not happiness that brings us gratitude.*
> *It's gratitude that brings us happiness.*
>
> — ANONYMOUS

QUESTION #1: "I am grateful for_____, because _____."

_____

_____

_____

QUESTION #2: "What am I looking forward to today (or tomorrow)?"

_____

_____

_____

QUESTION #3: List 10 things you like about your job or work-place.

_____

_____

_____

_____

_____

_____

_____

_____

DATE_____/_____/_____

> *It's not happiness that brings us gratitude.*
> *It's gratitude that brings us happiness.*
>
> — ANONYMOUS

QUESTION #1: "I am grateful for_____, because _____."

_____

_____

_____

QUESTION #2: "What am I looking forward to today (or tomorrow)?"

_____

_____

_____

QUESTION #3: List 10 things you like about your job or work-place.

_____

_____

_____

_____

_____

_____

_____

DATE_____/_____/_____

It's not happiness that brings us gratitude.
It's gratitude that brings us happiness.

— ANONYMOUS

QUESTION #1: "I am grateful for_____, because _____."

_____

_____

_____

QUESTION #2: "What am I looking forward to today (or tomorrow)?"

_____

_____

_____

QUESTION #3: List 10 things you like about your job or work-place.

_____

_____

_____

_____

_____

_____

_____

Final Thoughts on Gratitude

Congratulations on completing
The 90-Day Gratitude Journal.

You have dedicated the last ninety days to focusing on positivity, instead of surrounding yourself with negativity. Even if you've only journaled for a few minutes daily, you have discovered what it's like to recognize the good in the world.

Embracing gratitude can have a transformative effect on your life. As mentioned before, learning how to be more grateful will:

- Increase your happiness.
- Improve your mental health.
- Allow you to savor every positive experience.
- Help you cope with major life challenges.
- Create a sense of resilience in how you approach challenging experiences.
- Boost your self-esteem.
- Foster empathy for others.
- Provide a better night's sleep.
- Strengthen both your personal and romantic relationships.

After journaling for the past ninety days, you've probably experienced many of the benefits of gratitude. Not only is it a great habit that improves your life, it can also have a positive spillover effect on the people around you.

Now, we encourage you to frequently reread this journal—at least once a month. This practice will act as a reminder about all the amazing things that you have *right now*—not in some distant, faraway future.

Finally, we would love to hear about your experience with this journal, and which prompts you found most useful. If you'd like to share your thoughts feel free to email us at sjcott@developgoodhabits.com or support@barriedavenport.com

Thanks for investing both your time and money in *The 90-Day Gratitude Journal*.

We hope you enjoyed the journey of discovering unique ways to apply gratitude your daily life.

Cheers,

Made in the USA
Las Vegas, NV
07 August 2021